Power Walking and Foot Care

Take Walking

and Care for the Feet
Carrying You

to the Next Level

RON KNESS

Contents

Power Walking – Picking Up the Pace 1

Benefits of Power Walking 3

Power Walking Success Tips 5

Equipment Needed for Effective Power Walking 7

Dealing with Diabetes Foot Problems 10

Plantar Fasciitis 21

Common Foot Problems 30

Other Health and Fitness Books by This Author 39

About the Author 47

Power Walking – Picking Up the Pace

You're probably wondering what Power Walking is, and what is different from just regular old walking. Well, for one, with Power Walking you perform exaggerated walking movements. It doesn't have a very high impact on your feet.

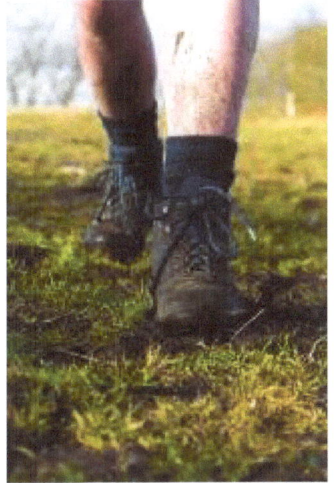

Secondly, you do it very fast without running. So, it's like running except you don't pound your joints like you do with running.

Finally, it's a fun, doctor-recommended form of exercise that almost anyone can do no matter their physical condition at the time. Within a short period of time from when you start power walking, you'll start looking better and feeling better.

Basically, in order to "Power Walk" you simply walk the way you normally do, except you need to exaggerate every move. Lift your knees up a little higher, push your arms back and forth a little more as if you need them to propel you, keep your spine straight, squeeze your glutes, and hold your stomach in and walk quickly.

It looks a little funny, but it's a great way to get fit. It's easier on your joints than jogging, but burns about the same amount of calories. Moving your arms back and forth causes your heart rate to go up higher than if you put them down to your side.

To challenge your body even more, carry a light set of hand weights or barbells. Lifting your knees causes your body to work a little harder.

When you power walk, the point is to make every single movement burn as many calories as possible. That's why you walk a little faster, move your arms back and forth a little higher and faster – to take advantage of the efficiency of your own body to get healthy and lose weight.

Benefits of Power Walking

Funny looking or not, power walking is a fun way to get your heart rate up, build muscle, and burn fat. There are many benefits to power walking that you may not have considered.

- **Help Manage Your Weight** – When you burn more calories you can lose more weight. Adding power walking to your day will make all the difference in whether or not your diet works.
- **Improve Your Heart Health** – Keeping your heart rate up will help you improve your cardiovascular health. Plus it will help you burn more calories which will help you get rid of dangerous stomach fat that is related to stroke and heart attacks.
- **Lower Your Stress Levels** – Exercising helps you keep your stress down. Power walking will lower stress levels so much because it's also fun since it looks so silly and is so easy to do.
- **It's Easy To Do** – With power walking you can get a great workout without having to do anything special. All you're doing is walking. No special equipment or skill needed.
- **No Special Equipment Needed** – Other than a good pair of walking shoes and comfortable clothing you don't need to go out and spend a lot of money on equipment. However there is that option should you decide to do so.
- **Any Age Group Can Do It** – If you can walk, you can power walk. You don't need to be fit to start. It's a great type of exercise for someone who is not yet fit to start with.

- **Fun to do alone or With a Group** – Power walking can be done alone, or with a group. Since all age groups can do it, you can get started power walking with your family.
- **Improve Your Mood** – Endorphins help you feel good and you will produce a lot when you start power walking. Try interval training for an even bigger metabolic boost.

Power walking is easy to do, fun to do, and very effective in helping with weight loss and improving cardiovascular health. Anyone who can walk, of all ages, can join in on the fun of power walking.

Power Walking Success Tips

In order to get the most out of power walking, take the time to get the right shoes and learn good posture. Learn the best way to carry your body and move your legs and arms that work for you to avoid causing neck, back and leg pain.

- **Wear the Right Shoes** – It's very important to ensure that the shoes you find are a good fit. They should be light weight, breathable, and fit correctly. It might help to get fitted for your first pair of walking shoes 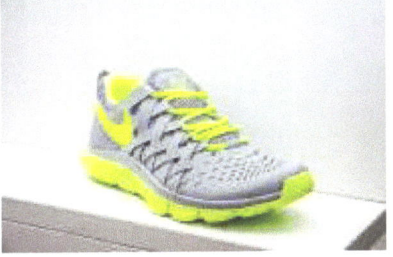 professionally. That way you can be sure that they fit right. Shoes that fit will help you walk comfortably, longer.
- **Warm Up** – Like with any exercise, warming up will help prevent you from injuring yourself. You can warm up with a few stretches and slow walking before you get into your power walk.
- **Use Good Posture** – Stand up straight, look ahead, pull in your belly and squeeze your bottom. This will ensure that you get the right type of exercise for each part of your body.
- **Engage Your Core** – One of your most important muscle groups reside in your core or your belly. Having a large round belly is an indicator of potential heart and cardiovascular disease but having a tight core is a sign of health.

To increase core health, practice holding your core taunt and firm as you power walk.

- **Swing Your Arms** – As you walk, try swinging your arms with your steps to help propel yourself forward and work your arm muscles. This will increase the effectiveness of your work out exponentially.
- **Be Natural** – Even though you're squeezing your glutes, swinging your arms, and engaging your core, you still want to try to be as natural as possible so that you don't injure yourself by forcing a position that doesn't work.
- **Set Goals** – If you have a goal that you want to achieve through power walking, whether it's distance, time, or weight loss you can do it. Ensure that any goals you set are realistic and actually can be done. Otherwise, you'll set yourself up for failure.
- **Boost Your Results** – Speed up for a minute at a time to get your heart pumping then go slow for four minutes. Keep doing this throughout your power walk session and you'll find that the results you want to achieve will happen even faster.
- **Cool Down** – Always take the time to cool down at the end of your power walk so that you don't get sore muscles or cramps. The cooling down process can simply involve slower walking until you stop sweating and your pulse is back to normal.

The most important tip of all is to keep your head up high and try to enjoy your walks. When you power walk, you'll start feeling energetic and wonderful within a week or two. Within a couple of months you'll have lost weight and improved your life exponentially.

Equipment Needed for Effective Power Walking

The great thing about power walking is that very little equipment is needed. You just need good shoes, clothing with comfortable moisture wicking fabrics, and if you really want to, you can use a pedometer or Fitbit and an iPod for music to boost your energy while you power walk.

Types of Shoes – Try on shoes to ensure a comfortable fit but get shoes that breathe to avoid itchy feet, and that support good posture in order to avoid lower back pain.

- A good shoe for women is the Skechers Women's Power Walking Shoe.
- For men the Skechers Sport Men's Skech-Flex Power Alley Oxford is a good walking shoe.

Moisture Wicking Clothing – When you wear clothing that takes away the sweat and keeps your body dry you can avoid rashes and other uncomfortable circumstances. There are a few choices that you might want to try to keep you comfortable when you walk.

For Women:

- Women's Short Sleeve Moisture Wicking Athletic Shirts - http://amzn.to/1OQKpiF, by Opna
- Women's Mid-Weight Wicking Thermal Leggings - http://amzn.to/1YJQ2iY, by Duofold

For men:

- DRI-EQUIP Long Sleeve Moisture Wicking Athletic Shirts - http://amzn.to/1XocyiG - by Joe's USA
- Men's Moisture-Wicking Mesh Reversible Spliced Shorts - http://amzn.to/1OQKt24, by Joe's USA

Electronics

Today there are a lot of electronics that you can use to make power walking more fun and to track your progress.

- Kamor Running Belts / Exercise Runner Belt / Waist Packs - http://amzn.to/1XocEqw – Help keep your phone safe and listen to podcasts while you're walking.
- Fitbit Charge HR Wireless Activity Wristband - http://amzn.to/1OQL18f – This can help you keep track of your steps.
- Apple iPod touch 16GB Blue - http://amzn.to/1WHnXf7 – Listen to music while you walk to help you keep up the pace.

Power walking is a fun way to burn fat, get fit, and see nature. You can do it alone, or with a group. It doesn't matter. You don't need fancy equipment either. You just need to get moving.

To get started, buy some shoes that are light-weight and comfortable to wear so that you'll want to wear them and walk often. Some moisture wicking clothes would be great too. You can get them online or even at department stores like Target and Walmart.

Set some goals, and try to commit to at least 30 days of Power Walking so you can see some real benefits develop from power walking before you choose to continue or not. Changes are, you'll lose weight, feel better and want to stick to your new exercise routine.

If you would like to learn more about developing a walking fitness plan, check out my book Design Your Ultimate Fitness Program – Walking (https://www.createspace.com/5252272).

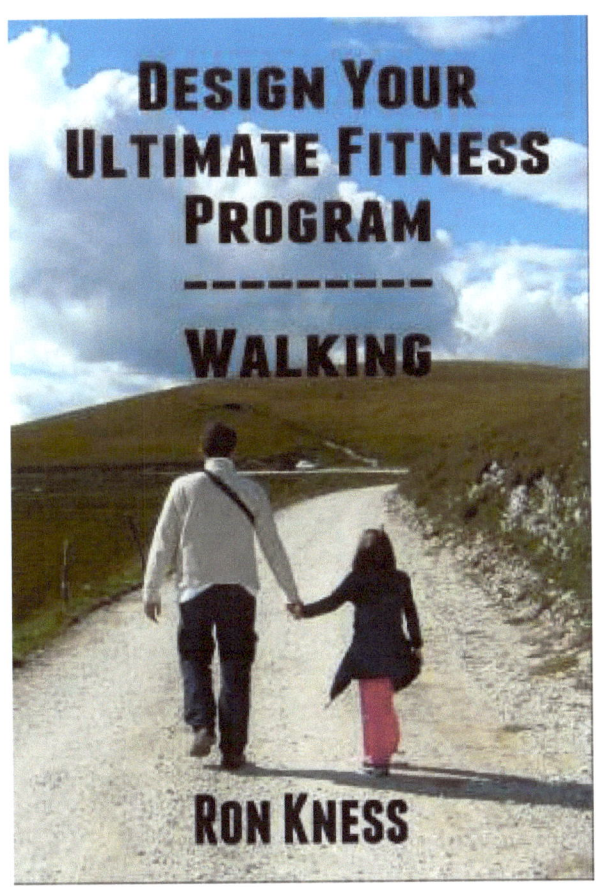

Or my other book on walking in the Kindle electronic format – *Walking Down the Road to Fitness*

(https://www.amazon.com/Walking-Down-Road-Fitness-Healthy-ebook/dp/B00PD8B6ES).

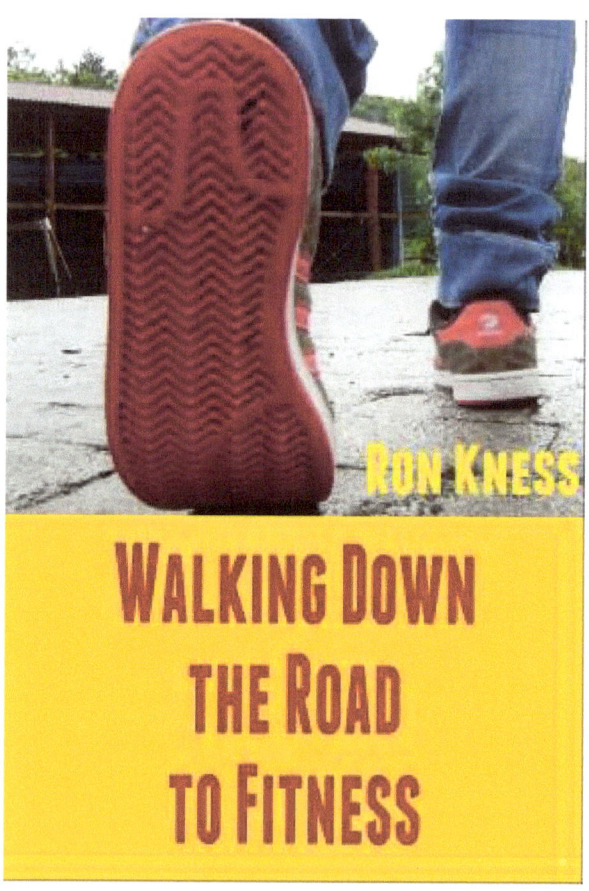

Dealing with Diabetes Foot Problems

Diabetes is known for being the worst disease that can do damage to your feet. There are two types of diabetes, Type I and Type II.

Type I is normally related to juvenile diabetes and is often a hereditary disease. The Type II is more usually known as adult diabetes and is common in people who are overweight and is characterized by high blood sugar levels.

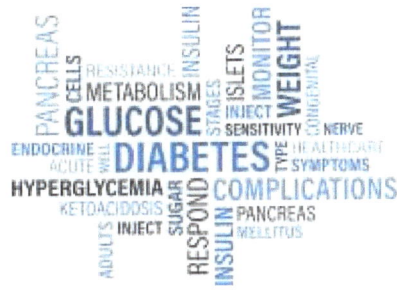

There is also a pre-diabetes condition also known as Syndrome-X and this is related to high blood pressure levels, people having a high BMI and high cholesterol level often develop this form. This type can also be associated with the onset of neuropathy, which is the loss of feeling or a tingling sensation in the feet and hands.

The most common foot problem that a person with diabetes can have is in developing foot ulcers. These ulcers will develop on the plantar or bottom of the foot. This occurs because the person cannot feel the bottom of their foot, when a sore develops it often goes untreated and can develop into a serious ulcer or infection. If this becomes really bad then losing a limb becomes a real possibility.

Treating foot problems is the major concern here. Your family doctor or podiatrist will work to relieve the pressure on your foot, along with preventing any serious infections from developing.

It is really important as a diabetic patient to take care of your feet. Wearing a good pair of diabetic shoes and socks, possibly along with diabetic insoles is one of the best ways to prevent foot problems from even starting.

A simple way to take care of your feet is to keep your feet clean, washing with warm water and soap every day. Many diabetic patients enjoy using foot spas and these can prove to be really therapeutic. Diabetics may not have good nerving endings in their feet and can easily burn themselves by using hot water.

Athletes' foot is another condition which is common in someone suffering from diabetes. If you are suffering from this it is best to change your shoes every other day. Doing this allows lots of time for your shoes to dry out completely. If you don't have a pair of diabetes socks, then wear cotton socks which are absorbent as well as applying foot powder daily.

Taking steps to improve your circulation is a huge help in ensuring your feet stay healthy. Massage your legs and feet daily to improve circulation. Even foot boots are very useful and inexpensive.

By taking proper precautions you can keep your foot health in top shape and not have to worry about developing dangerous diabetes foot problems including sores and ulcers.

Diabetes Foot Complications

Suffering from diabetes basically means that your glucose level is too high. This, however, can lead to other serious problems including foot and skin problems. Along with this diabetics can also suffer from heart and kidney disease, 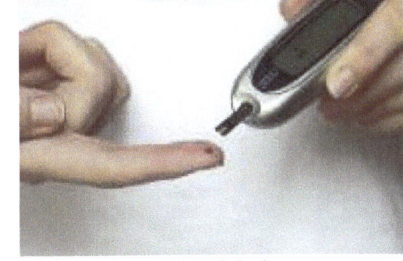 strokes, and eye damage. The problem most widely associated with diabetes is those from foot complications.

The two main reasons for diabetes foot problems are from diabetic neuropathy, this is where your nerve endings become damaged and you cannot feel sensations in your feet properly. This allows cuts and infections to go unnoticed for longer periods of time before treatment is administered.

The next reason is from peripheral vascular disease, this affects the blood flow going away from your heart and can have serious effects on your circulatory system.

What can happen from either of the two reasons mentioned above is that an injury does not receive the correct blood flow and tissue repair from your body. The tissue ends up dying and this is when the possibility of amputation comes into play. Because diabetic patients do not feel an injury, it is not noticed until it becomes a serious health risk. By this time it can be too late for treatment and the loss of a limb is imminent.

The risk of foot complications can be easily reduced just by taking better care of your feet. This includes getting regular checkups every two to three months.

Many foot problems can quickly lead to a more serious condition and these include suffering from any of the following:

- Athletes' foot

- Fungal infections

- Plantar warts

- Corns

- Calluses

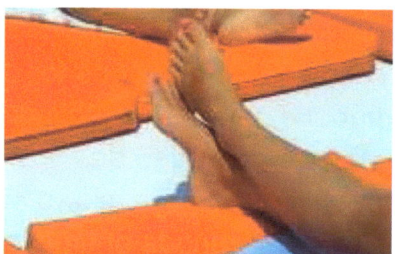

- Blisters

- Bunions

- Dry feet

- Foot ulcers

- Hammertoes

- Ingrown toenails

For people who don't suffer from diabetes these conditions are easily treated, though often uncomfortable and frustrating to deal with. For the diabetic patient they can all lead to severe problems if left untreated.

If you notice any signs of discoloration, swelling, pain in your legs, smelly foot odor or any condition that suddenly appears, then you want to seek medical advice immediately. Make it a habit to check your feet daily and to wash them with warm water. A good moisturizing foot lotion helps to alleviate dry skin, caused by poor circulation.

Using a foot spa or home massage system can also help keep your feet in great condition. A little bit of extra care can go a long way in avoiding diabetes foot complications from occurring in the first place.

Diabetic Foot Care

Having diabetes can be really dangerous for your feet. Maintaining a daily foot care regimen will be the best prevention method you can possibly do. Suffering from diabetes can mean that your nerves are damaged and your blood circulation is poor. What this entails is that you do not have proper feeling in your feet and even a slight cut can lead to serious side effects. Many people with diabetes have ended up losing a toe, foot or even a leg.

What this comes down to is understanding that taking extra precautions is extremely important for your diabetic foot care health. Keeping your feet in tip top condition is a matter of checking your feet more often. Each day you want to check

your feet for cuts, blisters and any abnormal looking redness. If you have trouble bending your feet up, use a small mirror to see the bottom of your feet properly. Any time you notice 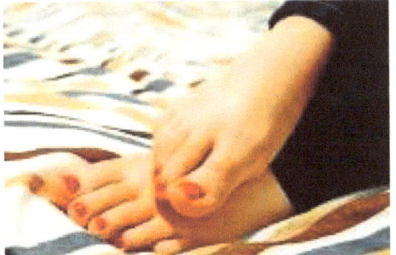 anything out of the ordinary be sure to set up a doctor's appointment right away.

As a diabetic your foot nerve endings might be damaged, this is why it is recommended that you always use warm water to soak your feet and not hot.

Wash your feet gently with a mild soap, baby soap is perfect to use. Pat your feet dry, do not rub or cause any excessive abrasions.

Using a good quality natural foot care lotion will help your skin stay soft, just don't put the lotion in between your toes as this might encourage a fungal infection. Wear a clean pair of socks each day and many doctors now recommend using diabetic socks. These are great especially if your feet tend to get cold during the night. Make sure your socks are not too tight so they don't restrict your circulation.

Before you put your shoes on in the morning always check them inside to make sure that they are dry and that there are no stones inside. Preventing any type of sore or cut is crucial to your foot care health. When you are at home always wear slippers around the house and don't walk barefoot. Again prevention is your aim here.

The diabetic food care routine described here is easy to follow and will effortlessly become a habit in a short amount of time. Along with your new routine just taking proper care of your diabetes overall will keep you healthy. Make sure your sugar levels are correct and always take the time to get regular checkups with your doctor or health care practitioner.

Why Diabetic Shoes are Worth the Money

Anyone suffering from diabetes is prone to be at risk of developing neuropathy, which is losing the sensation in your feet, especially the toe area. Using diabetic shoes helps with this by allowing more room for your feet to breathe and to move around.

This in itself is less likely to cause rubbing and sores developing on either your toes or the soles of your feet.

It really is important to make sure that you don't develop ulcers which could become infected and be the cause of you losing one or more of your toes. Diabetic shoes are designed to prevent any foot injuries from happening in the first place. Plus these types of shoes are roomier and allow you to use special diabetic insoles if required. Diabetic shoes are normally wider and deeper than a regular shoe.

You don't need to have custom shoes made but you should consider getting your feet measured and fitted by a

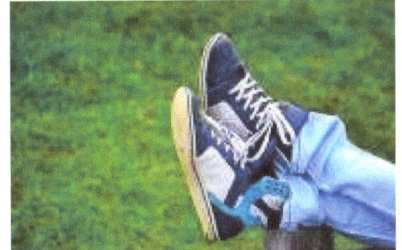

professional. Then you will be assured that your shoes will be comfortable and durable. A good quality pair of diabetic shoes will provide you with room for your foot, they will prevent pressure from building up while wearing your shoes. Plus they will be made of a breathable material. The toe area of the shoe will be wide and have plenty of room to allow your toes to move around.

The correct pair of diabetic shoe is going to make a world of difference to your comfort level. Some of these shoes are more expensive but many times will be covered in part by your medical insurance. If not you can find great deals on diabetic shoes online. Shoes such as therapeutic or medical shoes are often constructed in the same manner and are less expensive.

Always allow your shoes to dry out thoroughly and never wear them wet or without socks. If possible try not to wear the same pair of shoes each day and always check the inside of your shoe for pebbles or any type of debris, which could possibly damage your foot.

One of the easiest things to do to keep your feet healthy is to simply manage your diabetes better. Ensure that you are eating healthy, exercising appropriately and checking your blood sugar levels consistently.

Your feet carry you around all day and deserve a little extra tender care, whether you suffer from diabetes or not. Wearing diabetic shoes is a sure way to keep your feet in good condition and are well worth spending money on.

Why You Should Wear Diabetic Socks

One of the benefits of wearing diabetic socks is that they help to repel moisture away from your feet. This is especially important as diabetic patients are more likely to suffer from foot ulcers and pain more easily than those without diabetes.

A good quality diabetic sock is made without seams to prevent rubbing or chaffing. They are normally wrinkle free and this reduces the chances of blisters forming. Diabetic socks tend to be looser fitting around the top. This helps keep your blood circulation even and allows your foot to maintain its temperature.

Diabetic socks look no different to a regular pair of socks. They are made from a cotton blend and have a stretch top. Many manufacturers have come up with socks labeled as 'diabetic socks' and they do cost a little more. They come in various styles and colors.

Most doctors or podiatrists recommend wearing white socks if you currently have a foot injury. The reason for this is that you can easily tell on the white background if your wound is pussing or oozing.

Getting medical attention immediately is important for anyone suffering from diabetes, as foot injuries can quickly become a serious issue.

Keep the following in mind when purchasing your diabetic socks:

• **Moisture control** - the socks should be made of a high quality material, there are some new high tech fabrics on the market that help to keep moisture away better than cotton socks.

• **Reduce Pressure** – socks that have no seams are less likely to cause pressure on any part of your foot.

• **Reduce Wrinkles** – purchase socks which do not wrinkle, the wrinkles can cause irritations on your feet leading to blisters and foot ulcers. Avoid buying socks which are too thick and bulky.

• **Non-Binding** – your socks should not be too tight, as this could slow down or even stop your blood circulation. You want to choose socks which do not have elastic at the top, but will stay up by themselves.

• **Fitted socks** - these are usually more comfortable for diabetes sufferers as they will not bunch up as much. Try experimenting with a few styles to see what feels comfortable on your feet.

Diabetic socks really are the best solution for keeping your feet in excellent condition. As well as being more comfortable and lightweight, these socks are perfect for those with extra sensitive feet. Diabetic socks are found in most department stores alongside regular socks and can also be purchased online for extra shopping convenience.

I also have a couple books I have written on Diabetes management. One is titled How Diet and Exercise Can Better Manage Type 2 Diabetes.

It is available in either the Kindle or paperback formats at http://www.amazon.com/Diet-Exercise-Better-Manage-Diabetes/dp/1511510714 or just in paperback at: https://www.createspace.com/5404845.

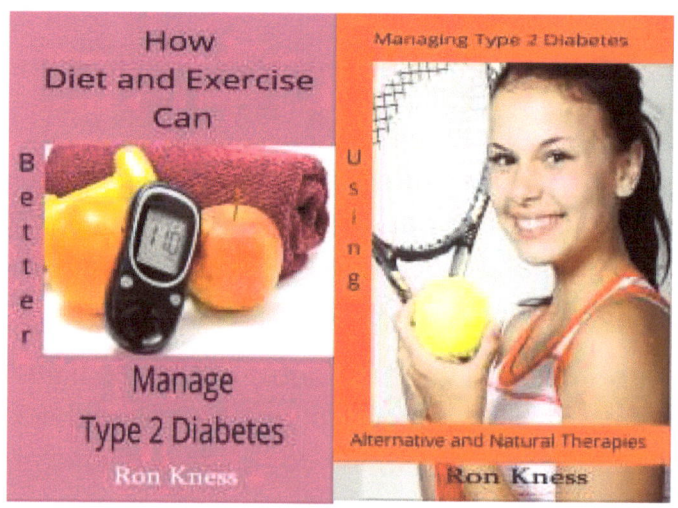

The other book – **Managing Type 2 Diabetes Using Alternative and Natural Therapies** in both Kindle and paperback is found at: https://www.amazon.com/Managing-Diabetes-Alternative-Natural-Therapies-ebook/dp/B00V76GVYU or in just paperback on CreateSpace at: https://www.createspace.com/5401244.

Plantar Fasciitis

Plantar Fasciitis is a common term heard very frequently these days. Millions of people are suffering from plantar fasciitis, with people in their fifties affected the most. This pain is felt in two sections of the foot, under the heel and in the back of the heel.

Plantar fasciitis occurs due to being overweight and from walking or standing on hard surfaces. However, the most common cause is by wearing ill-fitting shoes. It is extremely important to select a shoe which is the right size and the correct fit for your feet. Keep this in mind the next time you are out shopping for shoes.

Plantar Fascia is a thick tissue connecting your heal to the toes. It is the strong region of the foot which enables the foot to carry our weight and maintain balance. If the foot undergoes abnormal stress due to being overweight, or from walking or running for long 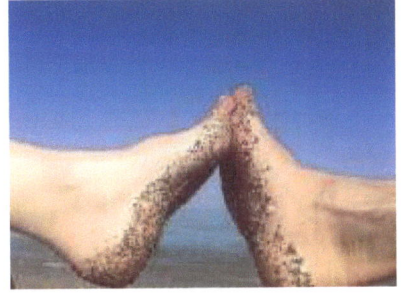 distances, it creates a tear in the planar fascia and causes pain.

Plantar fasciitis can be prevented effectively at home and is easy and inexpensive. Avoid doing long walks, running, jumping, or standing for long periods of time on hard surfaces. Avoid bare foot activities. Swimming is a good alternate exercise for running and walking.

Stretching your body and your muscles before doing any exercise is extremely important. you can do a soleus stretch or bicycle stretch. By stretching your body before walking or running, you can make plantar fascia flexible enough to minimize damage.

Maintaining healthy weight is very important to prevent plantar fasciitis. This will reduce the physical load on the plantar fascia.

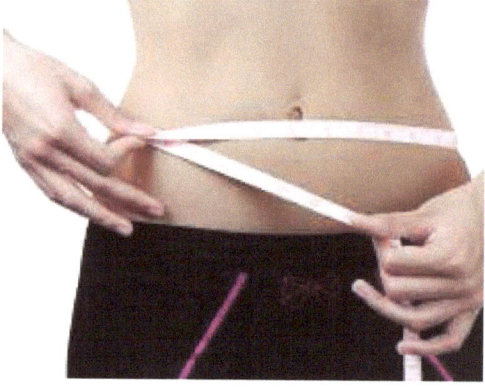

Reduce your weight by eating a healthy diet. Foods containing animal protein and fat such as beef, eggs and pork can be replaced by low fat healthy foods such as beans, nuts, lean chicken, vegetables, fruits.

Wearing appropriate shoes is also essential in preventing plantar fasciitis. Avoid using shoes which are completely flat and provide no foot support. Select a shoe which has a strong heel and good flexibility in the front and which allows the toes to move easily and naturally.

If you are using athletic shoes, replace them frequently. While shopping for shoes, keep in mind that finding shoes that offer support and cushioning is your highest priority. Massaging your feet with ice for 5-10 minutes can help relieve the pain to some extent.

If nothing works, surgery is an option. However, as there are complications involved in plantar fasciitis surgery, it should only be considered as a last resort.

Easy Ways To Treat Plantar Fasciitis

If you get up from the bed with foot pain, you might be experiencing plantar fasciitis. It is a condition where the tissues in the feet get damaged due to immense pressure applied on the heel. The pain starts slightly in the beginning and accelerates over time. It is particularly important to identify this condition and undergo plantar fasciitis treatment in the initial stage.

There are different methods to treat plantar fasciitis. Firstly, it is very important to give your heel ample rest. Avoid walking bare foot. Use the right size shoe to prevent pressure on the heel. It is no good to go for running or walking for long periods of time with this condition.

If you continue to walk while still in pain, it will aggravate the pain and make it tough to treat. Applying ice to the feet can be an enormous help. It will diminish the pain to a greater extent. If you cannot avoid walking or other activities, apply ice after you come home from walking. It will surely prevent the inflammation or pain from becoming too intense.

Exercise is an essential part of plantar fasciitis treatment. Simple exercises which can be done in the mornings and evenings, can give substantial relief to people affected with plantar fasciitis. Heel pain is most common while getting out of bed. If you experience heel pain, stretch your feet and flex your foot up and down 6-8 times.

If you have a tennis ball, try to roll your arch on the ball. Massaging in this way can release the tension on the fascia. Calf stretching is another exercise to release pressure on the feet. Place one leg forward and tilt your pelvis while holding the upper body upright.

Bend the knee until you feel the stretch on the other leg. Repeat this exercise about 10-12 times.

Hamstring exercises can also be done along with this exercise. Another method is to place marbles on the ground and pick them with your finger toes. Place them in a cup and repeat this action again. This releases the pain on the heel.

While you are asleep, the foot muscles are placed in the same position for a long time and cause pain when you get up in the morning. A night splint holds your foot flexed all night and prevents tightening of the plantar fascia. This will prevent the horrible pain you experience in the morning.

In addition, you can use oral medication or physical therapy. Surgery should be the last step in plantar fasciitis treatment. However, make sure that you wear the right shoes and avoid straining your feet to avoid plantar fasciitis.

Simple Yet Effective Tips To Treat Your Plantar Fasciitis

Plantar fasciitis exercises are not new for most people. People suffering from plantar fasciitis know how painful it is. Plantar fascia is a thick connecting tissue which supports the arch of the foot. If it undergoes immense pressure, the tissues tear out resulting in severe pain. It is commonly caused by wearing wrong shoes. Athletes and sports persons are more prone to it as they wear tight shoes and put pressure on the feet most of the time.

There are many ways to cure plantar fasciitis like oral medication, physical therapy or surgery. Plantar fasciitis exercises are a good way to reduce or prevent planar fasciitis in an effective manner.

However, make sure that these stretching exercises give you a pulling feeling and do not cause any pain.

If you experience foot pain while getting out of bed, a heel pain exercise is necessary to start your day out right. Plantar fascia gets tightened while you are asleep and you need to massage it. Stretch your foot and flex it up and down 8-10 times before getting up.

Try to roll a tennis ball with the arch so that the heel tissues get massaged. You can also perform this exercise while standing. It is recommended not to walk with bare feet as it puts immense pressure on the heel resulting in pain.

Calf stretch exercises can be done while standing. Turn towards the wall and place your hands on the wall. Place the leg you want to stretch, one step ahead. Bend one knee till you feel a stretch on the other leg. Keep it stretched for 15-20 seconds and release your legs. Repeat this exercise 4-5 times.

Another similar exercise is a hamstring exercise. While one foot is flexed, extend the other leg forward. Tilt your pelvis forward while keeping your body upright. Stay in that position for 15-20 seconds and feel the stretch at the back of the extended leg. Interchange the leg positions and repeat.

Using the stairs in your home is another easy exercise you can perform. Balance yourself on the balls of your feet. Slowly allow your body weight to stretch your calf muscle until you feel the stretch, hold this position for 30 seconds, then repeat.

When performing any Plantar fasciitis exercises stop if the pain is too much. You might only be able to perform one exercise once or twice. Work up to adding more repetitions daily. Your body has to adapt to any new exercise routine.

Discover How To Select The Right Shoes

Selecting the right size is very important when you are purchasing shoes. An ill-fitting shoe can get you into trouble. Plantar Fasciitis is a common phenomenon seen with people who wear badly fitting shoes. It is caused due to small tears formed at the heel bone. This is commonly seen in Athletes and sports people. It causes pain and discomfort while walking, running or any other movements involving your foot. Wearing appropriate shoes can prevent this ailment.

There are different ways to treat Plantar Fasciitis. The treatment varies with the severity of the problem. Many cases end up with surgery to enable free muscular movement. However, surgery is not recommended as there are many complications involved. Oral medication or physical therapy can be a good choice to reduce risks. You need to do regular exercises as advised by your doctor. Using Plantar Fasciitis shoes is another solution to reduce pain and prevent the growth of this disease.

Plantar Fasciitis shoes have become very popular in recent times. These shoes are commonly found everywhere. They are available in different models specifically designed for 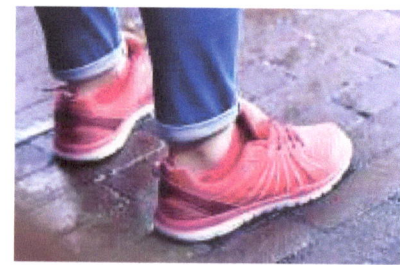 walking, running and for other movements.

Plantar fasciitis walking shoes are flat and have support in the heel area. The shoe allows the foot to move correctly and provides support to the arches. When purchasing shoes make sure that you are comfortable walking and that you can easily bend up and down while wearing them.

Plantar Fasciitis running shoes are specially designed to provide cushioning to your arches. While running, the entire weight of your body falls on your feet. In addition, gravitational forces and speed act on your foot. Therefore, you need to make sure that there is extra padding for your feet. This will minimize the pressure on your feet. With so many people suffering from Plantar Fasciitis, shoes are now available in great looking styles, no-one will know you are wearing a specialty shoe.

It is possible to customize your shoes to suit your style and comfort. Depending on your foot size and shape, you can order shoes. You need to be patient and choose the right shoe while shopping. If you are confused about what the right shoe is for you, you can contact a plantar fasciitis consultant. The consultant will measure and examine your feet and suggest the best brand for you.

Your feet are precious and spending money on shoes designed to relieve the pain of Plantar Fasciitis must surely outweigh the costs.

Learn About Different Types of Plantar Fasciitis Splints

A Plantar fasciitis splint is one of the best methods used to reduce foot pain. Plantar fasciitis is becoming more and more common these days. Plantar fasciitis treatment is available everywhere now.

There are many ways to treat this condition. Performing proper exercises, applying ice to that area or taking oral medication and physical therapy are some of the methods used to treat plantar fasciitis. However, a plantar fasciitis night splint can prevent the pain to a greater extent.

While you are asleep in the night, your planar fascia would be in the same position for a long time, and it gets tight. This is the reason for the pain in your foot when you get up in the morning. If you wear a plantar fasciitis night splint, it will hold the foot flexed and prevents the morning pain. A night splint holds your foot in a dorsiflexion position. The gentle stretching of this device reduces stress on your heel and enables the tissue to get back into its earlier length in due course.

There are different models of plantar fasciitis night splints available in the market. The most common splint is a boot night splint. The outer layer is made up of plastic while the inner region is soft and cushioned which gives more flexibility and a flexion angle of 10-30 degrees.

These splints are mostly used to reduce the pain at the back of the leg. Dorsel night splints are specially designed to reduce pain at the front of the leg. It contains straps to pull the toes upward. It is made up of foam core and a soft outer layer. Dorsel splints do not have any flexion angle and are exceptionally comfortable to wear during the night. They are light weight and are a comfortable shape to wear.

Sock night splints are available in different models, shapes and fabrics. They slip on like a sock, and the strap connected from the toes gives the flexion angle of 10 to 20 degrees. These are easy to wear and remove. They are made up of durable material and can be washed.

Sock night splints are also referred to as soft night splints. They reduce the stress on the heel and enable the tissues to get back to their normal length which reduces inflammation and pain.

If you read reviews from people who have used a plantar fasciitis splint, you will understand that these smaller devices are doing a fantastic job in reducing pain and restructuring foot tissues.

Common Foot Problems

Some of the most common foot problems include suffering from Plantar Fasciitis and this can turn into a very painful condition. Plantar Fasciitis normally occurs after undue pressure has been applied to the arch of the foot. Most sufferers will experience pain in the heel area which has become inflamed. Overnight your foot becomes stiff and getting out of bed in the morning can be very difficult indeed.

Bunions develop on the side of the big toe and turns into a fluid filled sac. The word bunion is also commonly used to describe a bony joint or deformity on the foot. Bunions normally occur due to wearing tight fitting shoes.

Neuroma is a condition where a nerve becomes irritated and becomes swollen. The longer the nerve stays inflamed and irritated the thicker the nerve becomes. The most common place to feel a Neuroma is on the ball of your feet.

Corns and Calluses often get confused, a corn develops due to being irritated and is always found on your toes. When you suffer from thick skin anywhere else on your foot it is known as a callous.

Your toenails are an ideal environment for fungus to grow, fungi love the dark, moist enclosure of your shoe. The fungus normally develops on your toenails and discolors them, the toenail can also become thick and loose.

Ingrown toenails occur when pressure on the nail forces it to grow inwards. If left untreated for any length of time the toenail can start to grow inside the skin. The area will become inflamed, red and very sore.

Another condition is called Hammer Toes and these form due to your foot tendons not working correctly. The tendon does not pull your toe correctly and eventually the toe curls up permanently.

Plantar Warts are caused by a virus infection and they can be very painful. Depending where on your foot they are located, you could experience discomfort when walking or even putting on your shoe.

Another fungus infection is Athlete's Foot and this is usually found on the bottom of your feet or in between your toes. The area can be red, itchy and have tiny blisters or peeling skin.

Achilles Tendonitis is a problem which if left untreated can develop into a permanent issue. If the Achilles tendon is allowed to stay inflamed for a long period of time, the tendon becomes very thick. In some people this tendon has been known to become ruptured.

If you are suffering from any of these common foot problems be sure to seek medical advice first. Many of these conditions can be treated with natural remedies and supplements found in many stores both on and off line. As well wearing a good quality shoe can ease your foot problems considerably.

Foot Treatment Regimen

Without the correct foot treatment regimen your feet will begin to undergo changes. You will start to suffer from sore feet and your skin will start to dry up. A little pampering will go a long way in keeping your feet healthy.

The worst case scenario is that you develop smelly feet and who wants to be known for having foot odor?

After a long day at work what is nicer than coming home and soaking your feet in some warm soapy water or maybe even in a foot spa. It is recommended that you soak your feet for no longer than 10 minutes. This is to prevent your skin from drying out excessively. Then pat your feet dry and massage some foot 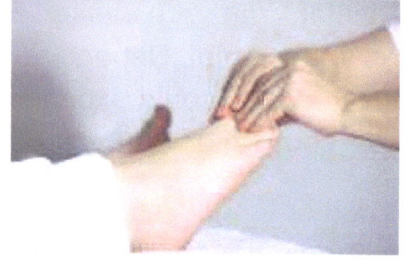 lotion into them. This will make your entire body feel relaxed and is a great way to re-energize after a hard day.

Sometimes we tend to forget about our feet and then wonder why we develop foot problems. Using a foot treatment regimen is an effortless way to ensure our feet stay healthy for years to come.

A Basic Foot Treatment Regimen:

•   Examine your feet weekly for any dry spots, blisters, calluses or anything that looks unusual.

•   Wash or soak your feet daily in warm water.

•   Pat your feet dry with a soft towel, don't rub as this can cause blisters.

•   Apply a good quality foot lotion.

•   Use powder if you suffer from sweaty feet.

•   Wear fresh socks each day.

• Always wear dry shoes and check for stones or debris before putting them on.

• Always cut your toe nails straight across.

When examining your feet, if you do notice anything unusual then check with your doctor. This is especially true if you suffer from foot pain which is relieved by taking the weight off of your feet. Other conditions to watch out for are tingling sensations in your feet that don't go away. Any injury that just doesn't want to heal and if 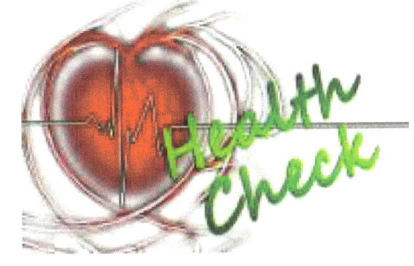 your foot or leg starts to turn black or blue for no apparent reason, these are all signs that medical attention is required.

Untreated foot pain can lead to many foot problems including plantar fasciitis, athlete's foot and other ailments. Our feet take a lot of stress each and every day, take the time to apply this basic foot treatment regimen and your whole body will thank you for it.

Natural Arthritis Treatment for your Achy Feet

Living with arthritis can be extremely difficult, suffering from this disease makes your joints achy and swollen almost every day. If you want to experience any degree of relief from arthritis then it is a good idea to look at an effective method of arthritis treatment for your feet.

There can be various reasons why you are suffering from arthritis, you possibly injured your feet many years ago and are now experiencing the consequences.

Consuming too much alcohol and being overweight are also reasons which result in arthritis. Any condition which suddenly breaks down large amounts of body tissue can be another cause.

You will know if you have arthritis in your feet as they will be sore and stiff after you have rested for any length of time. Standing or walking can cause pains in your feet or ankles. Your feet might hurt more with changes in the weather and the seasons. Another side effect is that your feet will become swollen and you may have a hard time moving your toes and flexing your ankle. All of this can make walking very difficult and extremely painful.

Your doctor will be able to determine if you have arthritis in your feet and unfortunately there is no cure for this. Arthritis treatment is done on an individual basis and you have to experiment to find what works for you the best.

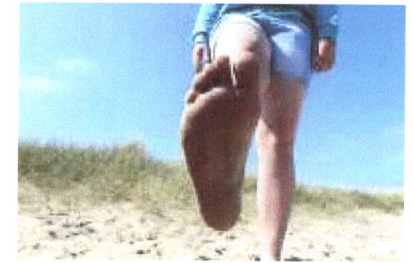

Keeping your weight under control is one easy way to alleviate the symptoms and pain of arthritis. Another way is to cut back or eliminate alcohol from your diet. Adding in some form of exercise each day will help to strengthen your muscles and will help to increase your flexibility. If your feet are your main cause of you looking for arthritis treatment then purchasing orthopedic shoes can help. These shoes will add support and comfort to your feet making walking more enjoyable.

Other forms of natural arthritis treatment include using supplements. The most common and the most effective of these is the use of Glucosamine and Chondroitin.

These two compounds can help in repair your joint tissue and keeping your joints healthy. Turmeric and Ginger are known to be anti-inflammatory herbs and have been proven to be extremely beneficial to arthritis sufferers.

As well there are many other combinations of natural supplements which can be used in your arthritis treatment. Using these as well as soaking and massaging your feet daily will help to provide you with a good level of relief. Your arthritis will be more manageable and less painful.

Using Glucosamine to deal with Foot Pain

There is nothing worse than having to suffer from excruciating foot pain whether it is your entire foot which is the cause of your pain, or you have heel pain. Looking for an effective treatment that actually works can be a long process. If your foot pain is severe then a checkup with your doctor can determine the cause of the problem.

No-one wants to take medications unnecessarily and many people prefer to look for natural remedies for their foot pain. With so many over the counter remedies how do you know which actually work and which act as nothing more than placebos?

If you do some research to find out what natural remedies work you will discover that there are various natural herbs which can help alleviate foot pain. These include the use of Glucosamine and Chondroitin, these substances are found naturally in your body and aid your body in protecting and healing your joints.

The thing to remember with these natural supplements is that you must take them on a regular basis. It normally takes about 2 – 3 weeks to start feeling the effects, then the person's foot pain will diminish within a couple of months and they stop taking their daily dose. Before they know it, the foot pain returns and they have to start the whole process over.

The whole key to reducing your foot pain is to reduce the amount of swelling in your feet, relieving your pain level and then slowing down the damage done to your joints. This is where you will benefit from taking Glucosamine. Glucosamine works by going straight to the area of your foot pain and starts work immediately. Your body's production of protein is stimulated, which assists the building and repair of your connective tissues.

As a person ages their body starts to produce less glucosamine so taking a daily supplement can be very beneficial in slowing down joint degeneration. Your body is able to handle good doses of this natural supplement but as with any herbal extract too much can have possible side effects. These would include nausea, skin rashes and heartburn.

When purchasing a brand of Glucosamine for your foot pain, look for a good quality supplement which has all the ingredients listed on the bottle. Cheaper brands may not have the high quality of ingredients and ultimately you will not get full benefits from your supplement.

Why Orthopedic Shoes are the Best Choice for your Feet

If you experience any type of foot or leg pain it can be difficult to walk around all day doing your daily routine.

If the pain you are experiencing is coming to a point where it is almost unbearable then you might want to consider purchasing a pair of orthopedic shoes. If you have a pre-existing medical condition then your health insurance should cover part of the cost of your orthopedic shoes.

Even so the expense of a new pair of shoes can be outweighed by the benefits. Once you have a shoe that fits your foot it will be so much more comfortable to walk. After you take your shoe off your foot will not be as sore and achy. Many people have noticed a decrease in their foot and knee pain within days of wearing a good pair of orthopedic shoes.

An orthopedic shoe is manufactured to fit your foot correctly and is made of high quality and breathable materials. Many times shoe inserts or insoles can be placed inside the shoe for added comfort. The toe section of an orthopedic shoe is wider than a normal shoe allowing more room for your feet to move. This is great for anyone suffering from swollen toes, hammer toes and other foot issues. Diabetic patients often wear these types of shoes to prevent pressure from building up and causing sores or calluses.

Manufacturers have replaced the once looking big and bulky orthopedic shoe with more stylish options. Today you would have a hard time distinguishing who was wearing an orthopedic shoe and who wasn't. With so many people having access to the internet, shopping for shoes online is a viable option and allows you to shop for bargain prices.

A good quality shoe will allow you to walk with no discomfort or pain. These types of shoes have good support for your arches and heels.

The breathable materials allow room for air to circulate around your foot, preventing toenail fungus from developing.

Arthritis sufferers also benefit from orthopedic shoes, the shoe will help lessen the impact of walking on their knees and hips. These joints are prone to be more susceptible to developing arthritis and osteoporosis as you age. Taking care of our joints in our younger years will prevent the likelihood of foot and knee problems from developing.

You have many options when shopping for a pair of orthopedic shoes, always ensure that you get your foot measured correctly and buy accordingly. A good pair of shoes can easily last you 6 months of more before they need replacing and the additional comfort is well worth the cost.

Other Health and Fitness Books by This Author

If you would like to read more about Senior Health and Fitness, here is a list of the <u>titles, CreateSpace links and descriptions:</u>

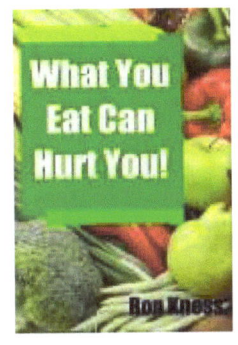

[What You Eat Can Hurt You](#)

https://www.createspace.com/4963196

Do you know that certain foods increase your risk for inflammation, disease and illness? It's true! And certain foods can help cure and heal you if you do get sick. Knowing which foods to eat and which ones to avoid empowers you to manage your own health.

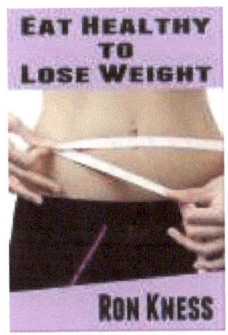

[Eat Healthy to Lose Weight](#)

https://www.createspace.com/4962939

As you read through our book, we show you which foods you should and should not be eating to reach your weight loss goal, along with discussing how to maintain your weight loss and stay within a few pounds of your goal weight. Banish the weight you keep gaining back each time by learning how to live a healthy lifestyle.

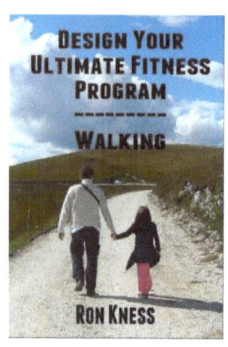

Design Your Ultimate Fitness Program - Walking

https://www.createspace.com/5252272

In my book Design Your Ultimate Fitness Program – Walking, we discuss the considerations that need to be made when designing a custom walking program, along with:
• Equipment needed
• Wearable technology you can use to track your walking
• And how to make walking more challenging

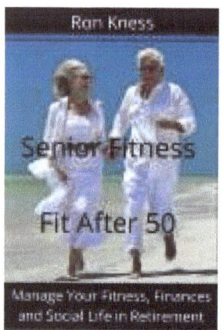

Senior Fitness – Fit After 50: Learn How to Manage Your Fitness, Finances and Social Life in Retirement

https://www.createspace.com/5474751

Inside you will discover answers to your most pressing questions:
• What do I need to know about downsizing my home?
• What are the best tips for staying healthy as you approach your 50's?
• When should I start planning for retirement?
• I am worried about being lonely once I retire, do others feel the same?
• Is it worthwhile to carry two homes during retirement?
And more…

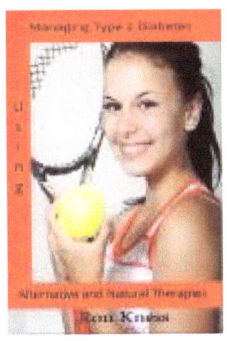

[Managing Type 2 Diabetes Using Alternative And Natural Therapies](#)

https://www.createspace.com/5401244

While Type 2 diabetes can be managed medically, there are many alternative natural and holistic methods of therapy and treatment that can further enhance quality of life and minimize the effects of this disease. In this book, I discuss 12 different types, including yoga, reflexology and acupuncture to name just three.

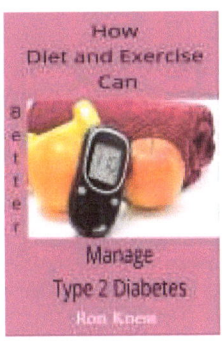

[How Diet and Exercise Can Better Manage Type 2 Diabetes](#)

https://www.createspace.com/5404845

Of the different types of diabetes, only Type 2 can be reversed. In my book How Diet and Exercise Can Better Manage Type 2 Diabetes, we reveal the three things you can do to best manage your disease, including:
• Diet
• Exercise
• Weight management

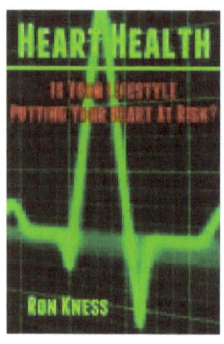

Heart Health: Is Your Lifestyle Putting Your Heart at Risk?

https://www.createspace.com/5464020

In my ebook Is Your Lifestyle Putting Your Heart At Risk? we discuss the six greatest risks to your heart and the lifestyle changes you can make to mitigate them.

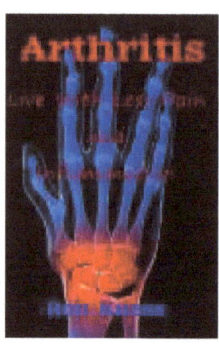

Arthritis – Live Wth Less Pain and Inflammation: Tips and Techniques You Can Use to Lessen the Pain and Inflammation

https://www.createspace.com/5457441

Discover Simple Tips & Information That Will Help Reduce The Painful Symptoms Of Arthritis!

You learn things like:
• Simple and effective information that will help you manage the pain and inflammation that comes along with arthritis, so that you can live an active, full life without debilitating pain.
• The different types of arthritis, their symptoms and how to alleviate their painful side effects.
• The pros and cons of over-the-counter arthritis medications, plus simple tips that will help you know how to choose the right supplements.
• Free, yet effective ways to get relief from arthritis pain and

inflammation, so you don't have to suffer anymore.
The effects arthritis can have significant impact on your physical and mental well-being, but this books shows you how to overcome its painful symptoms and live life relatively pain free.

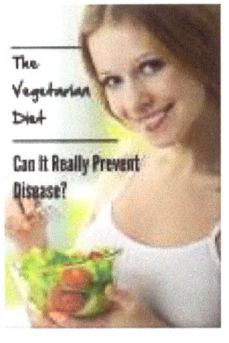

The Vegetarian Diet – Can It Really Prevent Disease?

https://www.createspace.com/5519874

Is a vegetarian diet right for you? Multiple studies have shown over and over that a vegetarian diet goes along way in preventing certain chronic diseases, such as:

- Heart Disease
- Cancer
- Diverticulitis
- Type 2 Diabetes
- Hypertension
- Obesity
- Kidney Failure

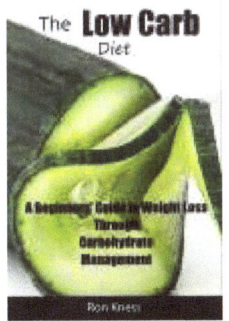

The Low Carb Diet: A Beginner's Guide to Weight Loss Through Carbohydrate Management

https://www.createspace.com/5416348

In my book "The Low-Carb Diet – A Beginners' Guide to Weight Loss Through Carbohydrate Management", I reveal a successful method of losing weight based in part on the amount and type of carbohydrates you consume.

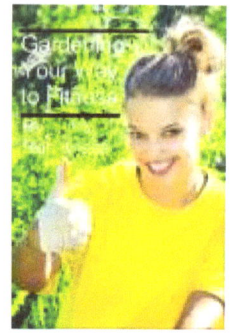

Gardening Your Way to Fitness: The Fun Way to Get Fit and Provide Beauty and Healthful Bounty for Your Family

https://www.createspace.com/5459564

The gym is a great place to stay fit during the colder seasons, but once the temperature turns warmer you want to spend more time outside. Plus, you'll have the benefit of fresh wholesome produce to enjoy by growing vegetables in your backyard garden.

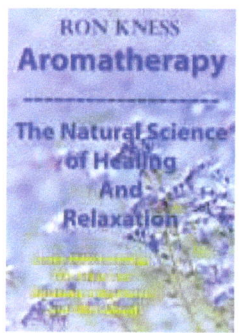

Aromatherapy - The Science of Healing and Relaxation: Learn How Essential Oils Elicit The Relaxation Response And Alter Mood

https://www.createspace.com/5714434

In my book Aromatherapy – The Science of Healing and Relaxation, we reveal the natural holistics methods you can use to heal the body from certain medical issues and to relive stress through relaxation. In particular we talk about:
• Aromatherapy - what it is and how it works

• Essential Oils – how the effects of certain aromas differs from others

• Recipes – how to make your own essential oil combinations

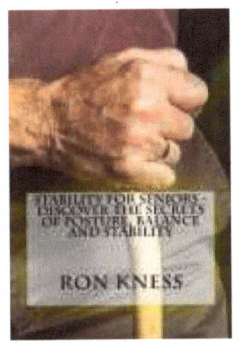

Stability for Seniors: Discover the Secrets of Posture, Balance and Stability

https://www.createspace.com/6096479

Many people sacrifice their health in pursuit of their career. They are so busy making a living that they neglect to make a life. The excuse that they do not have time to exercise is tossed about so frequently that they end up letting their health and fitness slide.

If you are not regularly active, you will have muscular atrophy over time. Your flexibility will decrease. Your core strength will diminish. As time progresses, you will be less limber and more rigid.

This is exactly how people age poorly. It's a process that has snowballed over time.

Only with regular exercise and a healthy diet can you have a body that is fit and has the ability to almost reverse aging.

If you have neglected your health for years and life seems to be a chore now because you can't get around without assistance, do not feel dejected.

You can remedy the situation. You can restore the strength,

balance and stamina that you have lost. It is never too late to become what you might have been.

This guide will show you exactly what you need to do to restore your balance, strengthen your core and give you the ability to live life to its fullest. Read how …

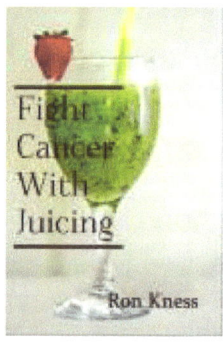

Fight Cancer With Juicing

https://www.createspace.com/6155567

Juicing is a healthy practice that has allowed millions of people to boost their nutrition. Juicing fruits and vegetables provides you important antioxidants, which scavenge for oxygen free radicals that can damage cellular structures, including DNA. When DNA is damaged, it can result in mutations that lead to cancer.

Well-balanced nutrition from a variety of healthy whole foods helps support and maintain on-going good health, and experts agree that nutrition plays a key role in preventing chronic and terminal illness.

Juicing is practiced by millions around the world and it is an easy and convenient way to get plant nutrition into the body to do its magic.

When juicing is done right, that is when the majority of your juice blends is comprised of vegetables and very low sugar fruit, you can easily boost your nutritional intake thereby improving your health and lower your risks for cancer.

About the Author

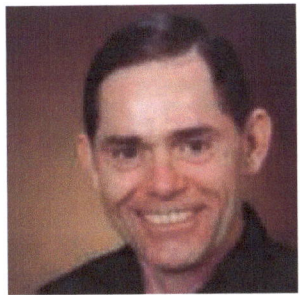 I grew up in Central Minnesota, where my parents own and operated a fishing resort. Once out of high school I tried a couple of semesters of college, only to quit halfway through the Spring term; I decided at that time that college wasn't for me.

Then I decided to follow my father's previous occupation as an auto mechanic. I graduated from a two-year of vocational training course and worked as a mechanic. While in vocational training, I decided to join the National Guard where I eventually ended up working full-time for 32 years.

So how does all of this relate to writing? In one of my leadership schools, the instructor, who was an English teacher at a juvenile detention center, presented writing to me in a whole new way - a way that started to develop my interest in working with words.

Fast forward about 40 years and I now have over 50 books listed on Amazon for Kindle and CreateSpace.